Trademark, Ownership, Intangible Property

In a letter dated March 27, 2014 the Secretary, Health and Human Services asserted ownership of the program (ideas) and the materials developed to disseminate the program. Further, in 2011, portions from the original Tai chi: Moving for Better Balance implementation guide, instructors' manual, supplemental materials, and participants' course book produced by ORI were adapted by the National Center for Injury Prevention and Control, and disseminated via the internet as "Tai chi Moving for Better Balance: A Guide for Program Implementation. The program and materials are presumed to reside in the public domain. -IPC

Soon after, the Guide disappeared. All references and links on government sites delivered the reader to a trademarked program, not the program owned by the government.

While researching the program, Ed. discovered the links before the blackout, and downloaded the file. The following pages are that file.

Additionally, Ed. has seperately developed materials for continuing education of physical and occupational therapists, and tai chi instructors. These materials are periodocally revised based on the outcome of various training evaluations. These materials are are provided as a separate volumn to this series,volumn 4.

Under federal law, the Department of Health and Human Services retains a royalty-free, non-exclusive and irreversible right to reproduce, publish, and otherwise use intangible property developed pursuant to awards. 45 C.F.R. §§ 74.2 & 74.36. This applies to the tai chi program that Dr. Li developed with HHS grant CE05-029. A primary purpose of that award was the development of a fall-prevention exercise program package "that can be delivered to community-based organizations for implementation with older adults."(Funding Opportunity Announecment NumberCE05-029 FedReg 64,76 Novemeber 8, 2004.)) -General Counsel for the HHS

Translation of an Effective Tai Chi Intervention Into a Community-Based Falls-Prevention Program Am J Public Health. 2008 July; 98(7): 1195–1198. doi: 10.2105/AJPH.2007.120402 FOA Number: CE05-029 - Dissemination Research on Fall Prevention: Development & Testing of an Exercise Program Package Project Period: 9/1/05-8/31/08 Application/Grant Number: 1-U49-CE000711-01

LJS-Ed.

Disclaimer

Reference herein to any specific commercial products, programs, or services by trade name, trademark, manufacturer, or otherwise, does not necessarily constitute or imply its endorsement, recommendation, or favoring by the United States Government. The views and opinions expressed are those of the authors and do not necessarily represent the official views of the U.S. Government or the Centers for Disease Control and Prevention, and shall not be used for advertising or product endorsement purposes.

REVISED 07/18

Table of Contents

Table of Contents	i
Introduction	iii
Section One: Roadmap to the T*ai chi: Moving for Better Balance* Guide	1
Section Two: *Not included in this volume*	3
Introduction to Tai chi	3
Overview of *Tai chi: Moving for Better Balance*	5
Administrative Preparation	7
Starting a Course	8
The Importance of Partnerships	10
Program Sustainability	13
Final Thoughts	14
Section Two Appendices: *Not included in this volume*	15
Section Three: *Not included in this volume*	32
About the Instructors' Guidebook	32
Tai chi: Moving for Better Balance Background Information	32
Course Logistics	34
Classes and Students	34
Warm-Up and Cool-Down Exercises	37
Core Tai chi Exercises	38
Teaching Considerations	40
Program Modifications	42
Information about Program Fidelity	42
Instructor Preparation	44

Pagination of the complete guide is maintained across all volumes. A student, instructor, or administrator only need to have their respective document (Vol III, Vol II, and Vol I). They will be able to discuss information referencing the same page numbers. -Ed.

Instructor Networking 44

Summary of Instructors' Guidebook 44

Section Three Appendices *Not included in this volume* 45

Section Four: *Tai chi: Moving for Better Balance* **Participants' Guidebook** . . . 53

Using the Participants' Guidebook 53

Background and Benefits of Tai chi 54

About the Eight-Form Tai chi 55

General Practice Guidelines 56

Recommended Practice Schedule 59

Section Five: *Tai chi: Moving for Better Balance* **Movements** 72

Form One: Hold the Ball 72

Form Two: Part the Wild Horse's Mane 77

Form Three: Single Whip 82

Form Four: Wave Hands like Clouds 86

Form Five: Repulse Monkey 90

Form Six: Brush Knees 94

Form Seven: Fair Lady Works at Shuttles 98

Form Eight: Grasp the Peacock's Tail 103

Put it All Together and Make it Flow 112

Key Resources 119

A companion *Tai chi: Moving for Better Balance DVD* is available at Amazon.com

Introduction

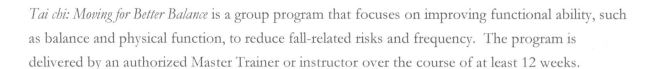

Tai chi: Moving for Better Balance is a group program that focuses on improving functional ability, such as balance and physical function, to reduce fall-related risks and frequency. The program is delivered by an authorized Master Trainer or instructor over the course of at least 12 weeks.

A team of researchers at the Oregon Research Institute (ORI) developed *Tai chi: Moving for Better Balance*, which was tested and demonstrated effective in decreasing the number of falls, the risk of falling, and fear of falling, and improving functional balance and physical performance among persons aged 70 and older.[1] The program uses eight forms that have been derived from the traditional 24-form Yang-style Tai chi, and progresses from easy to difficult.

While *Tai chi: Moving for Better Balance* is an effective intervention for fall prevention, the Centers for Disease Control and Prevention's (CDC), National Center for Injury Prevention and Control (NCIPC) acknowledges that *Tai chi: Moving for Better Balance* is one of many evidence-based interventions for the prevention of falls. In particular, CDC recognizes that the most effective and cost-effective of these interventions are those that combine fall risk assessments done in clinical care practice with targeted evidence-based exercise and home hazard reduction programs. Assessing an older adult in clinical care practice is seen as crucial prior to participation in an evidence-based exercise program.[2] Although *Tai chi: Moving for Better Balance: A Guide for Program Implementation* is one of the first evidence-based fall intervention guides to be introduced by CDC, it is of but many that will be promoted now and in the future.

To develop this compilation of *Tai chi: Moving for Better Balance* program materials, CDC consulted with public health experts from around the United States. The materials should be used with the program as it is disseminated and implemented throughout the United States. Program materials include:

- Portions from the *Tai chi: Moving for Better Balance* implementation guide, instructors' manual, supplemental materials, and participants' course book (produced by ORI and adapted by NCIPC),

- Input and feedback from state health department representatives and other partners who were involved in the pilot projects,

- Recommendations from the Safe States Alliance that conducted a multi-site evaluation of an initial pilot of *Tai chi: Moving for Better Balance* in four state health departments, and

- Sections and recommendations from CDC's publication, *Preventing Falls: How to Develop Community-based Fall Prevention Programs for Older Adults*, that provides guidelines to community-based organizations interested in developing effective fall prevention programs.

REVISED 7/18

Section One:
Roadmap to the Tai chi: Moving for Better Balance Guide

CDC provided a grant with which three guides were developed for implementing *Tai chi: Moving for Better Balance* throughout the United States. The guides outline the program and provide the needed direction for completing each of the program's eight forms of Yang-style Tai chi. These guides, compiled with additional information outlined in the *Introduction*, can be found in Sections Two through Five of this manual. Contact CDC at Falls-Prevention@listserv.cdc.gov for periodic updates to these guides.

Summary of *Tai chi: Moving for Better Balance* Compilation

- **Implementation Plan.** Designed for organizations such as state health departments, local senior centers, and area agencies on aging.
- **Instructors' Guidebook.** Designed for individuals who have been trained by authorized Master Trainers to instruct program participants.
- **Participants' Guidebook.** Designed as an in-home practice guide for older adults practicing *Tai chi: Moving for Better Balance*.
- ***Tai chi: Moving for Better Balance* Movements.** Designed for implementers, Master Trainers, instructors, and participants to use as they teach and learn the program's movements.

Detailed descriptions of each guide and a section that describes each Tai chi movement are provided below. Note that portions of each of the sections designed to be used by older adults have larger size print. CDC recommends font sizes between 12 and 14 points to ensure readability by older adults.[3]

- ***Tai chi: Moving for Better Balance* Community Implementation Plan**
    - Section Two includes the Community Implementation Plan which provides information about *Tai chi: Moving for Better Balance* to implementing organizations. It includes the background and benefits of the program, how to set up each class, the materials that are needed by both the Master Trainer or instructor and the program participants, how to plan for and promote the course, how to ensure the safety of program participants, and how to

monitor and evaluate the program. The Appendices provide sample forms that implementers can use if they so wish. Examples include an attendance sheet and a physical activity readiness questionnaire.

- ***Tai chi: Moving for Better Balance* Instructors' Guidebook**
  - Section Three includes the Instructors' Guidebook which provides *Tai chi: Moving for Better Balance* instructors with the teaching elements of the program. It was designed for instructors who had been trained by either the developer of the program, Fuzhong Li, PhD, or a Master Trainer. The guidebook provides an overview and information about the importance of the program and the essential elements of the course (e.g., duration and frequency, sequence of the eight forms, proper breathing). It also describes how to make program modifications, gives information about in-class and at-home exercises, and provides evaluation forms.

- ***Tai chi: Moving for Better Balance* Participants' Guidebook**
  - Section Four includes the Participants' Guidebook which gives program participants information to support their Tai chi home practice and reinforces what was learned at each class session. The Participants' Guidebook is a compilation of the information in the Users' Guidebook and the Step-by-Step Guide developed by Fuzhong Li, PhD. It gives participants background on Tai chi, particularly as it relates to research evidence and health outcomes and describes safe ways to practice the movements at home. The Participants' Guidebook also provides a recommended at-home practice schedule for each of the 12 weeks, including frequency and duration of practice, the forms to practice, the number of forms to be practiced in one session, the number of repetitions per form, and warm-up and cool-down exercises. The Participants' Guidebook may be supplemented by the *Tai chi: Moving for Better Balance* DVD that was created to guide participants in their at-home practice. Contact the Oregon Research Institute to obtain the DVD (contact information on page six).

- ***Tai chi: Moving for Better Balance* Movements**
  - Section Five gives program implementers, Master Trainers, instructors, and participants step-by-step instructions about how to execute the movements needed to complete each of the eight Tai chi forms. Pictures of each movement are provided along with verbal cues on how to perform each movement appropriately and safely.

Section Three:
Tai chi: Moving for Better Balance Instructors' Guidebook

About the Instructors' Guidebook

This guidebook gives instructors a brief but comprehensive overview of the essential elements involved in teaching the *Tai chi: Moving for Better Balance* program. Available at Amazon.com

Section Four:
Tai chi: Moving for Better Balance Participants' Guidebook

- By participating in this exercise program, you have chosen to learn and practice a style of Tai chi that has been specifically developed for older adults, is easy to follow, and is fun to do.
- *Tai chi: Moving for Better Balance* is designed to improve older adults' balance, reduce their chances of falling, and help them improve and maintain their mobility, functional independence, and quality of life well into their later years.
- *Tai chi: Moving for Better Balance* is the result of years of scientific research and practical workshops conducted with older adults living in the community.
- *Tai chi: Moving for Better Balance* is a simplified Tai chi program consisting of just eight individual forms.
- The key to mastery is to practice each form individually as often as possible. Once you are confident in performing each form, they can be linked together into a flowing sequence.
- This guidebook and the DVD are designed to complement and reinforce your *Tai chi: Moving for Better Balance* classes. You may find it valuable to use the *Tai chi: Moving for Better Balance* DVD that was created to guide participants in their home practice. The DVD may be obtained by contacting the Oregon Research Institute.

Using the Participants' Guidebook

This guidebook and the companion DVD are designed for those who take part in the *Tai chi: Moving for Better Balance* program.[33,34] It is offered as support for your home practice and to reinforce what you learn in class. This allows you to gain as much from the program as possible by helping you to practice whenever you like.

We recommend that you watch the DVD once or twice to get an overall impression of what the eight Tai chi forms look like and how they are structured before you begin your home practice.

The instructions contained in this guidebook will help you remember how to practice the forms, first one by one, and later as a linked sequence. This guidebook is meant to supplement the group exercise program led by a Tai chi instructor. It may be used in conjunction with classes and/or home practice after completing classes. For best results, we recommend that you study and practice the forms in the order they are presented.

In this guidebook, you will find information about Tai chi and this program, including:

- Background and Benefits of Tai chi,
- About the Eight-Form Tai chi,
- General Practice Guidelines, and
- Recommended Practice Schedule.

Background and Benefits of Tai chi

Origins of Tai chi

The ancient Chinese practice of Tai chi has its origins in the martial arts. It combines combative elements (e.g., pushing and pulling, attacking, and yielding) with powerful healing qualities using one's "vital energy" or *Qi* (pronounced chee). One legend suggests that Tai chi was derived from observations of animal movements. Postures best suited for combat were created. This may explain why many Tai chi forms include animals in their names (e.g., Grasp the Peacock's Tail).

What is Tai chi?

Tai chi is a series of individual dance-like movements (or forms) that flow smoothly from one form to another in a sequence. When it is performed, Tai chi synthesizes elements of movement, mind and meditation, making it a mind-directed moving exercise.

Health-Related Benefits

Studies have shown that older adults experience many health benefits from practicing Tai chi. These include:

- Improved functional balance and physical performance,
- Reduced frequency of falls and risk of falling,

- Lowered blood pressure,
- Improved mental and physical well-being,
- Improved cardiovascular and respiratory function,
- Improved sleep quality, and
- Enhanced life independence and overall health.

How Tai chi Promotes Balance

Long-term practice of Tai chi improves balance. When you perform Tai chi you respond to gentle demands on your posture's stability. This low-intensity program improves strength and balance.

Problem of Falls among Older Adults

One in three people age 65 and older falls each year and 20 to 30 percent of people who fall suffer moderate to severe injuries, such as bruises, hip fractures, and head traumas. Falls are the leading cause of injury and deaths among older adults.

Research Evidence

Studies have shown that Tai chi improves muscular strength, balance, and postural control. Older adults who practice Tai chi are half as likely to fall as people of similar age who do not exercise.

About the Eight-Form Tai chi

In Brief

In the late 1990s, researchers at the Oregon Research Institute began to evaluate the health benefits of Tai chi for older persons. Over the years, they have scientifically demonstrated the efficacy of Tai chi, using the standard 24-form Yang styles, in improving older adults' balance and physical functioning. Based on their findings, they developed this exercise program tailored to older adults who want to improve their balance and mobility.

This program's focus is on preventing falls. Tai chi, when practiced regularly, will improve older adults' balance and reduce their chances of falling. The eight single forms in the program are derived from the traditional 24-form Yang-style Tai chi but are tailored to community adults.

Movement Characteristics

- **Number of movements:** There are eight forms in this Tai chi routine. These forms are largely derived from the traditional 24-Form Yang-style Tai chi that was developed by experts from ancient Chinese exercise forms.
- **Movement basics:** All forms adhere to the fundamental principles of traditional Tai chi and involve weight-bearing and non-weight-bearing stances, correct body alignment and posture, and multiple coordinated movements executed in a continuous, circular, and flowing manner. The performance of the forms is closely synchronized with natural breathing. Each movement coordinates with the breathing cycle, inhaling deeply through your nose and exhaling through your mouth.
- **Movement sequence:** The eight single forms are arranged in a sequential order, following a progression from easy to more difficult. Each of these forms can be performed and practiced repeatedly as a single movement or in combination as part of a routine.

General Practice Guidelines

Important reminder: As with other exercises, always begin with warm-up exercises before practicing Tai chi.

Warm-Up Exercises

Before each practice session, begin with basics, such as light walking, stretching, and deep breathing. Simple Tai chi-based exercise movements are also strongly encouraged. Warm-up exercises include:

- Walking in place to warm-up major muscle groups – one minute,
- Stepping sideways (one or two steps on each side) – five to six times per side,
- Single steps forward (right leg leads, followed by left leg) – two times each leg, and
- Gently stretching arms and legs.

Building up Your Practice Routine Over Time

- Focus initially on practicing and repeating individual forms.
- Once you feel confident about performing all the forms, link all eight forms into a sequence.
- Increase the health benefits by practicing the routine from form 1 through form 8 and then backwards from form 8 to form 1, making it a continuous loop.

A Word about Breathing

- Deep breathing is an integral part of Tai chi. However, emphasis on deep breathing in the early stages of learning and practice can be an unnecessary distraction.
- In general, breathing should be done naturally and go with your practice rhythm.
- As a general rule, inhale deeply through your nose as you extend your arms outward or upward and exhale through your nose as you contract your arms or bring them downward.

Cool-Down Exercises

Examples of cool-down exercises include:

- Repeating some of the warm-up exercises listed above.
- Standing quietly with arms raised to shoulder level, then lowering your arms to the side. Inhale as you raise your arms and exhale as you lower the arms. Perform these movements as many times as needed.

Safety Tips

Prevent injury and control body posture during each of your practice sessions by following these safety tips:

- If you have any doubt about your physical condition, stop practicing Tai chi. Discuss your condition with your primary care provider before starting the Tai chi program.
- If you have a history of knee problems or arthritis, modify your stance and bend your knees comfortably to reduce pressure on your knees.
- Always begin a practice session with warm-up exercises and end with cool-down exercises as previously indicated.
- Always take small or comfortable steps when performing each movement. Place your lead foot lightly on the floor to prevent foot injuries and be aware of your knee-to-toe alignment.

Important Notice Regarding Personal Health

Consult your primary care provider before engaging in the Tai chi program shown in the DVD and described and pictured in the accompanying printed instructions. Do not do any part of the program if it conflicts with your provider's advice and recommendations.

The forms should be adapted to your unique circumstances and physical limitations. Do the exercises without straining so you will not injure yourself.

Important Notice Regarding Liability

- People who engage in the activities described in this program do so at their own risk.
- The creators and distributors of this program do not assume any liability from the use of this guidebook, the DVD, or from performing any of the Tai chi forms.
- This program is not a substitute for medical care.

Recommended Practice Schedule

Here is the recommended home practice schedule for 12 weeks. Use this to help plan your practice and gradually build on the skills learned in class as you continue to do Tai chi each week. Keep track of the number of times you practice each week by checking (X) in the Completed Box (☐) of the form below.

In each of the weekly schedules, focus on frequency (how often), duration (how long), specific forms (which form to practice), and repetitions (how many times you repeat each form).

Frequency: In accordance with the U.S. Surgeon General's Guidelines, we encourage you to practice at least five days a week, including the time spent in class.

Duration: You will want to start with five minutes per practice session and slowly work your way towards 25–30 minute sessions by week 12. Each day the practice session will get longer and emphasize additional forms and repetitions.

Forms to practice: Practice one or two forms per session, working up to eight forms by the eighth or ninth week. The forms to be practiced at each session and for each week are indicated (see alphabetical key).

Number of repetitions per form: Practice each single form eight to ten times.

Number of forms to be practiced in one session: The number of forms that you should link together and practice as a whole sequence. This varies from week one to week twelve, as indicated.

Check the box on the day you did the exercise: Please put a check in the box below the day you completed the exercise. This allows you to keep track of the number of times you practiced each week and to see whether you have met the general exercise guidelines.

Week One Schedule

Goal: Learning and performing TWO forms:

a. "Hold the Ball," and
b. "Part the Wild Horse's Mane."

Frequency:	Day 1	Day 2	Day 3	Day 4	Day 5
Duration:	5–8 minutes	5–8 minutes	8–10 minutes	10–12 minutes	10–12 minutes
Forms to practice:	a	a	a, b	a, b	a, b
Number of repetitions per form:	5 to 8	5 to 8	5 to 8	8 to 10	8 to 10
Number of times forms are being practiced sequentially:	3	4	5	6	6
Check the box on the day you exercised:	☐	☐	☐	☐	☐

You have made a good start. Congratulations! You are now ready to move on to WEEK TWO.

Class Notes

Week Two Schedule

Goal: Performing and refining the TWO forms learned previously and also learning and performing Form Three:

a. "Hold the Ball,"
b. "Part the Wild Horse's Mane," and
c. "Single Whip."

Frequency:	Day 1	Day 2	Day 3	Day 4	Day 5
Duration:	10–12 minutes	10–12 minutes	12–15 minutes	12–15 minutes	12–15 minutes
Forms to practice:	a, b	a, b	a, b	a, b, c	a, b, c
Number of repetitions per form:	8 to 10	8 to 10	8 to 10	10 to 12	10 to 12
Number of times forms are being practiced sequentially:	4	5	5	6	6
Check the box on the day you exercised:	☐	☐	☐	☐	☐

Another week! Give yourself a hand to congratulate yourself. You are now ready to move on to **WEEK THREE.**

REVISED 07/18

Class Notes

Week Three Schedule

Goal: Performing and refining the THREE forms learned previously and also learning and performing Form Four:

a. "Hold the Ball,"
b. "Part the Wild Horse's Mane,"
c. "Single Whip," and
d. "Moving Hands like Clouds."

Frequency:	Day 1	Day 2	Day 3	Day 4	Day 5
Duration:	12–15 minutes	12–15 minutes	15–18 minutes	15–18 minutes	15–18 minutes
Forms to practice:	a, b, c	a, b, c	a, b, c	a, b, c	a, b, c
Number of repetitions per form:	10 to 12	10 to 12	10 to 12	12 to 15	12 to 15
Number of times forms are being practiced sequentially:	3	4	5	6	6
Check the box on the day you exercised:	☐	☐	☐	☐	☐

Another week! Give yourself a hand to congratulate yourself. You are now ready to move on to WEEK FOUR.

Class Notes

REVISED 07/18

Week Four Schedule

Goal: Reviewing and practicing the FOUR forms learned:

   a. "Hold the Ball,"
   b. "Part the Wild Horse's Mane,"
   c. "Single Whip," and
   d. "Moving Hands like Clouds."

Frequency:	Day 1	Day 2	Day 3	Day 4	Day 5
Duration:	15–18 minutes	15–18 minutes	15–18 minutes	18–20 minutes	18–20 minutes
Forms to practice:	a, b, c, d	a, b, c, d	a, b, c, d	a, b, c, d	a, b, c, d
Number of repetitions per form:	12 to 15	12 to 15	12 to 15	15 to 17	15 to 17
Number of times forms are being practiced sequentially:	3	4	5	6	6
Check the box on the day you exercised:	☐	☐	☐	☐	☐

You are doing great! Keep up the good work! You are now ready to move on to **WEEK FIVE**.

Class Notes

Week Five Schedule

Goal: Reviewing and practicing the FOUR forms learned previously and also learning Form Five:

a. "Hold the Ball,"
b. "Part the Wild Horse's Mane,"
c. "Single Whip,"
d. "Moving Hands like Clouds," and
e. "Repulse Monkey."

Frequency:	Day 1	Day 2	Day 3	Day 4	Day 5
Duration:	18–20 minutes	18–20 minutes	20–25 minutes	20–25 minutes	20–25 minutes
Forms to practice:	a, b, c, d	a, b, c, d	a, b, c, d	a, b, c, d, e	a, b, c, d, e
Number of repetitions per form:	15 to 17	15 to 17	15 to 17	17 to 20	17 to 20
Number of times forms are being practiced sequentially:	3	4	4	4	4
Check the box on the day you exercised:	☐	☐	☐	☐	☐

Just great! Now you are really showing progress! You are now ready to move on to WEEK SIX.

Class Notes

Week Six Schedule

Goal: Reviewing and practicing the FIVE forms learned previously and also learning Form Six:

a. "Hold the Ball,"
b. "Part the Wild Horse's Mane,"
c. "Single Whip,"
d. "Moving Hands like Clouds,"
e. "Repulse Monkey," and
f. "Brush Knee."

Frequency:	Day 1	Day 2	Day 3	Day 4	Day 5
Duration:	20–25 minutes	20–25 minutes	20–25 minutes	20–25 minutes	20–25 minutes
Forms to practice:	a, b, c, d, e	a, b, c, d, e	a, b, c, d, e	a, b, c, d, e, f	a, b, c, d, e, f
Number of repetitions per form:	8 to 10	8 to 10	8 to 10	8 to 10	8 to 10
Number of times forms are being practiced sequentially:	3	4	4	4	4
Check the box on the day you exercised:	☐	☐	☐	☐	☐

Well done again! This is really good! You are now ready to move on to **WEEK SEVEN**.

Class Notes

Week Seven Schedule

Goal: Reviewing and practicing the SIX forms learned previously and reinforcing Form Six:

a. "Hold the Ball,"
b. "Part the Wild Horse's Mane,"
c. "Single Whip,"
d. "Moving Hands like Clouds,"
e. "Repulse Monkey," and
f. "Brush Knee."

Frequency:	Day 1	Day 2	Day 3	Day 4	Day 5
Duration:	20–25 minutes	20–25 minutes	20–25 minutes	20–25 minutes	20–25 minutes
Forms to practice:	a, b, c, d, e, f	a, b, c, d, e, f	a, b, c, d, e, f	a, b, c, d, e, f	a, b, c, d, e, f
Number of repetitions per form:	8 to 10	8 to 10	8 to 10	8 to 10	8 to 10
Number of times forms are being practiced sequentially:	4	5	5	5	5
Check the box on the day you exercised:	☐	☐	☐	☐	☐

Excellent! You have now covered three-quarters of the whole sequence! You are now ready to move on to WEEK EIGHT.

Class Notes

Week Eight Schedule

Goal: Reviewing and practicing the SIX forms learned previously and learning Form Seven:

a. "Hold the Ball,"
b. "Part the Wild Horse's Mane,"
c. "Single Whip,"
d. "Moving Hands like Clouds,"
e. "Repulse Monkey,"
f. "Brush Knee," and
g. "Fair Lady Works at Shuttles."

Frequency:	Day 1	Day 2	Day 3	Day 4	Day 5
Duration:	20–25 minutes	20–25 minutes	20–25 minutes	20–25 minutes	20–25 minutes
Forms to practice:	a, b, c, d, e, f	a, b, c, d, e, f	a, b, c, d, e, f, g	a, b, c, d, e, f, g	a, b, c, d, e, f, g
Number of repetitions per form:	8 to 10	8 to 10	6 to 8	6 to 8	6 to 8
Number of times forms are being practiced sequentially:	5	5	3–4	3–4	3–4
Check the box on the day you exercised:	☐	☐	☐	☐	☐

Great progress! Keep up the good work! You are now ready to move on to WEEK NINE.

Class Notes

Week Nine Schedule

Goal: Reviewing and practicing the SEVEN forms learned previously while mastering Form Seven:

a. "Hold the Ball,"
b. "Part the Wild Horse's Mane,"
c. "Single Whip,"
d. "Moving Hands like Clouds,"
e. "Repulse Monkey,"
f. "Brush Knee," and
g. "Fair Lady Works at Shuttles."

Frequency:	Day 1	Day 2	Day 3	Day 4	Day 5
Duration:	20–25 minutes	20–25 minutes	20–25 minutes	20–25 minutes	20–25 minutes
Forms to practice:	a, b, c, d, e, f, g	a, b, c, d, e, f, g	a, b, c, d, e, f, g	a, b, c, d, e, f, g	a, b, c, d, e, f, g
Number of repetitions per form:	6 to 8	6 to 8	6 to 8	6 to 8	6 to 8
Number of times forms are being practiced sequentially:	3–4	3–4	3–4	3–4	3–4
Check the box on the day you exercised:	☐	☐	☐	☐	☐

Wow! Your confidence and mastery are starting to show. You are now ready to move on to WEEK TEN.

Class Notes

Week Ten Schedule

Goal: Reviewing and practicing the SEVEN forms learned previously and learning Form Eight:

a. "Hold the Ball,"
b. "Part the Wild Horse's Mane,"
c. "Single Whip,"
d. "Moving Hands like Clouds,"
e. "Repulse Monkey,"
f. "Brush Knee,"
g. "Fair Lady Works at Shuttles," and
h. "Grasp the Peacock's Tail."

Frequency:	Day 1	Day 2	Day 3	Day 4	Day 5
Duration:	20–25 minutes	20–25 minutes	20–25 minutes	20–25 minutes	20–25 minutes
Forms to practice:	a, b, c, d, e, f, g	a, b, c, d, e, f, g	a, b, c, d, e, f, g	a, b, c, d, e, f, g, h	a, b, c, d, e, f, g, h
Number of repetitions per form:	6 to 8	6 to 8	6 to 8	4 to 6	4 to 6
Number of times forms are being practiced sequentially:	3–4	3–4	3–4	2–3	2–3
Check the box on the day you exercised:	☐	☐	☐	☐	☐

Nearly there! You have almost completed all eight forms! You are now ready to move on to WEEK ELEVEN.

REVISED 07/18

Class Notes

Week Eleven Schedule

Goal: Reviewing and practicing the EIGHT forms learned previously while mastering Form Eight:

a. "Hold the Ball,"
b. "Part the Wild Horse's Mane,"
c. "Single Whip,"
d. "Moving Hands like Clouds,"
e. "Repulse Monkey,"
f. "Brush Knee,"
g. "Fair Lady Works at Shuttles," and
h. "Grasp the Peacock's Tail."

Frequency:	Day 1	Day 2	Day 3	Day 4	Day 5
Duration:	30 minutes	30 minutes	30 minutes	30 minutes	30 minutes
Forms to practice:	a, b, c, d, e, f, g, h	a, b, c, d, e, f, g, h	a, b, c, d, e, f, g, h	a, b, c, d, e, f, g, h	a, b, c, d, e, f, g, h
Number of repetitions per form:	4 to 6	4 to 6	4 to 6	4 to 6	4 to 6
Number of times forms are being practiced sequentially:	2-3	2-3	2-3	2-3	2-3
Check the box on the day you exercised:	☐	☐	☐	☐	☐

Well done! Your confidence and achievement are there for all to see! You are now ready to move on to WEEK TWELVE.

Class Notes

Week Twelve Schedule

Goal: Reviewing and practicing ALL EIGHT forms learned previously while mastering the whole routine:

a. "Hold the Ball,"
b. "Part the Wild Horse's Mane,"
c. "Single Whip,"
d. "Moving Hands like Clouds,"
e. "Repulse Monkey,"
f. "Brush Knee,"
g. "Fair Lady Works at Shuttles," and
h. "Grasp the Peacock's Tail."

Frequency:	Day 1	Day 2	Day 3	Day 4	Day 5
Duration:	30 minutes	30 minutes	30 minutes	30 minutes	30 minutes
Forms to practice:	a, b, c, d, e, f, g, h	a, b, c, d, e, f, g, h	a, b, c, d, e, f, g, h	a, b, c, d, e, f, g, h	a, b, c, d, e, f, g, h
Number of repetitions per form:	4 to 6	4 to 6	4 to 6	4 to 6	4 to 6
Number of times forms are being practiced sequentially:	2–3	2–3	2–3	2–3	2–3
Check the box on the day you exercised:	☐	☐	☐	☐	☐

Congratulations! You've made it through! Consider having a celebration with your classmates – you deserve it! Remember to keep up your practice and make Tai chi a part of your daily routine – you've worked hard to learn it so – use it, don't lose it!

REVISED 07/18

REVISED 07/18

Section Five:
Tai chi: Moving for Better Balance Movements

Form One: Hold the Ball

STEP 1

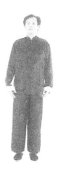

Step 1: Stand straight with feet slightly apart, knees unlocked, arms relaxed at the side of the body, and elbows slightly bent.

STEP 2

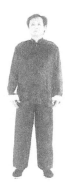

Step 2: Step slowly to your left with your left foot (toes touch down first, ending with feet spaced shoulder width apart).

STEP 3

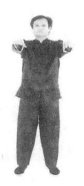

Step 3: Slowly raise both arms, with the elbows slightly bent, to shoulder height, wrists relaxed, hands dropped.

STEP 4

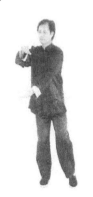

Step 4: Gradually shift your body weight to the right while dropping your left arm across your torso to the right. Have both palms face each other to form the first "hold the ball" position (beach ball size) on the right.

STEP 5

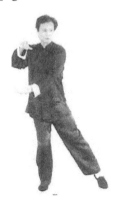

Step 5: Take a small and comfortable side step with your left foot directly to the left.

STEP 6

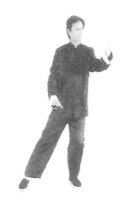

Step 6: Slowly shift your weight onto your left leg, allowing the left arm to move away from your body and upwards to your left (palm faces the body about eye level) while pushing the right hand down to stop at your right hip.

STEP 7

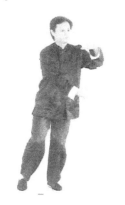

Step 7: Move your right foot close to the left foot while turning your left wrist over (palm faces down) and move the right hand across the lower body to take a position under the left hand (check: the palms of your two hands are now facing each other again forming a second "hold the ball" position on the left).

Now repeat Steps 5 to 7 on the right side.

STEP 8

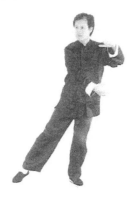

Step 8: Take a small and comfortable side step with your right foot to your right.

STEP 9

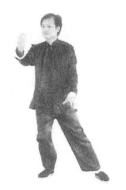

Step 9: Slowly shift your weight onto your right leg, allowing the right arm to move away from your body and upwards to your right (palm faces the body about eye level) while pushing your left hand down to stop at your left hip.

STEP 10

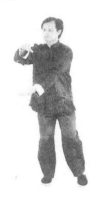

Step 10: Move your left foot near the right foot (shoulder width apart). While turning your right wrist over, move the left hand across the lower body to take a position under the right hand (check: the palms of your two hands are now facing each other again forming a "hold the ball" position on your right).

STEP 11

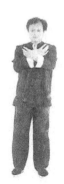

Step 11: Bring both arms to the front crossing them at the wrists with palms facing you.

STEP 12

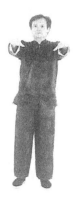

Step 12: Extend both arms forward allowing them to separate at shoulder level (check: palms face down).

STEP 13

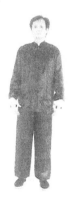

Step 13: Lower both arms to your side.

STEP 14

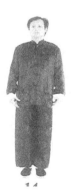

Step 14: Draw your left foot to your right to close the form.

Form Two: Part the Wild Horse's Mane

STEP 1

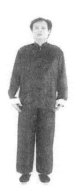

Step 1: Stand straight with feet slightly apart, knees unlocked, arms relaxed at the side of the body, and elbows slightly bent.

STEP 2

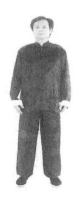

Step 2: Step slowly to your left with your left foot (toes touch down first, ending with feet spaced shoulder width apart).

STEP 3

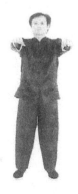

Step 3: Slowly raise both arms, with the elbows slightly bent, to shoulder height, wrists relaxed, hands dropped.

STEP 4

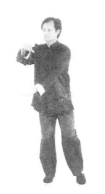

Step 4: Gradually shift your body weight to the right while dropping your left arm across your torso to the right to have both palms face each other to form the first "hold the ball" position (beach ball size) on the right.

STEP 5

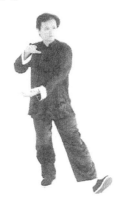

Step 5: From the "hold the ball" position, your left foot steps diagonally forward 45 degrees (heel lands first).

STEP 6

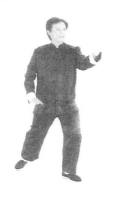

Step 6: Move your weight forward onto your left leg. At the same time, move your left arm up to about eye level (palm faces you). Your right hand pushes downward over the left wrist (as if you are stroking a horse's mane) to stop next to your right hip.

STEP 7

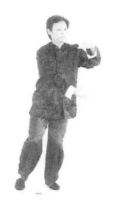

Step 7: As your rear foot moves up and beside the left foot, turn right palm up and move it under the left hand so both arms form a "hold the ball" position on the left.

Now repeat Steps 5 to 7 on the right side.

STEP 8

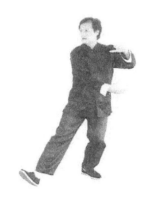

Step 8: To continue, step your right foot diagonally forward 45 degrees (heel lands first).

STEP 9

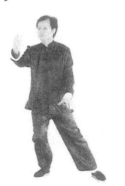

Step 9: Move your weight forward onto your right leg and sweep your right arm up to about eye level (palm faces you). Your left hand pushes downward over your right wrist (as if you are stroking a horse's mane) to stop next to your left hip.

STEP 10

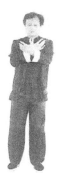

Step 10: As your left (rear) foot moves up and beside your right foot, bring both arms together to cross the wrists in front of your chest (check: your weight should be evenly balanced on both feet).

STEP 11

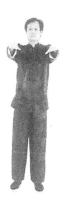

Step 11: Extend both arms forward allowing them to separate (check: palms face down) at shoulder level.

STEP 12

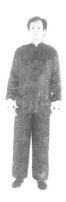

Step 12: Lower both arms to your side.

STEP 13

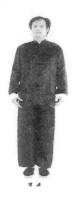

Step 13: Move your left foot near your right (shoulder width apart) to close the form.

Form Three: Single Whip

STEP 1

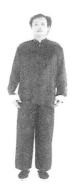

Step 1: Stand straight with feet slightly apart, knees unlocked, arms relaxed at the side of the body, and elbows slightly bent.

STEP 2

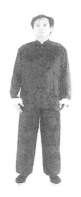

Step 2: Step slowly to your left with your left foot (toes touch down first, ending with feet spaced shoulder width apart).

STEP 3

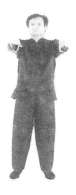

Step 3: Slowly raise both arms, with the elbows slightly bent, to shoulder height, wrists relaxed, hands dropped.

STEP 4

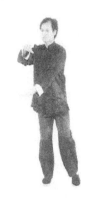

Step 4: Gradually shift your body weight to the right while dropping your left arm across your torso to the right to have both palms face each other to form the first "hold the ball" position (beach ball size) on the right.

STEP 5

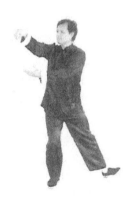

Step 5: With your weight still on your right leg, take a small and comfortable step slightly backward to your left and with your extended right hand form a hook (hand dropped at wrist, thumb touching all four fingers).

STEP 6

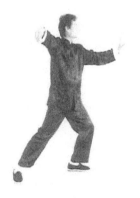

Step 6: Pivot on your left heel about 90 degrees, slowly rotate your trunk to your left, allowing your left hand to follow your trunk rotation and then turn the wrist and extend it palm outwards.

STEP 7

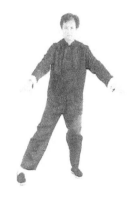

Step 7: Shifting weight to the right, pivot on your left heel (90 degrees) to the front, and at the same time, drop both arms.

STEP 8

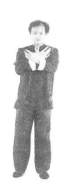

Step 8: Now, shift weight to your left foot, bring your right foot beside your left foot, shoulder width apart, and raise both arms up to your chest level, allowing the wrists to cross in front of your chest (check: your weight is now centered).

STEP 9

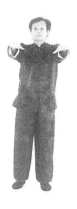

Step 9: Extend both arms forward, allowing them to separate (check: palms face down) at shoulder level.

STEP 10

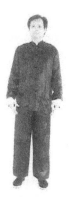

Step 10: Lower both arms to your side.

STEP 11

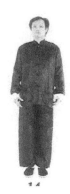

Step 11: Move your left foot near your right (shoulder width apart) to close the form.

PROGRAM NOTE: *There are no movements to the right.*

Form Four: Wave Hands like Clouds

STEP 1

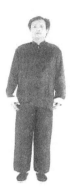

Step 1: Stand straight with feet slightly apart, knees unlocked, arms relaxed at the side of the body, and elbows slightly bent.

STEP 2

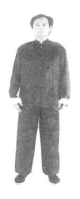

Step 2: Step slowly to your left with your left foot (toes touch down first, ending with feet spaced shoulder width apart).

STEP 3

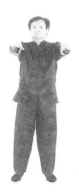

Step 3: Slowly raise both arms, with the elbows slightly bent, to shoulder height, wrists relaxed, hands dropped.

STEP 4

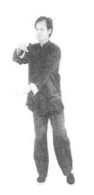

Step 4: Gradually shift your body weight to the right while dropping your left arm across your torso to the right to have both palms face each other to form the first "hold the ball" position (beach ball size) on the right.

STEP 5

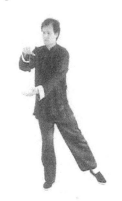

Step 5: Take a small and comfortable sidestep (slightly backward) to your left.

STEP 6

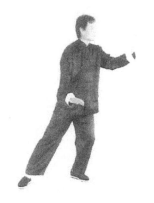

Step 6: Slowly shift your weight onto your left leg by rotating your trunk in the same direction. At the same time, move your left (leading) hand up (eyes following this leading hand) to the left about eye level (palm faces inward), allowing the right (trailing) hand to follow naturally to the left, but at a lower level (palm faces down).

STEP 7

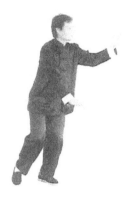

Step 7: Draw the right leg next to the left leg (feet shoulder width apart).

STEP 8

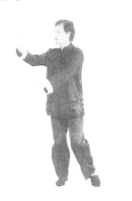

Step 8: Turn your torso again to the right with weight slowly transferring to your right; simultaneously, move your right (leading) hand upward to the right (eyes following this leading hand) about eye level (palms facing inward), allowing the left (trailing) hand to follow naturally, but at a lower level (palm faces down).

Now, repeat the movements described in Steps 5 through 8 twice. After completing Step 8, do the following:

STEP 9

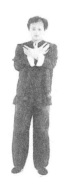

Step 9: Bring both arms to the front, crossing them at the wrists with palms facing you.

STEP 10

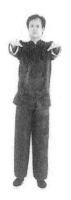

Step 10: Extend both arms forward allowing them to separate (check: palms face down) at shoulder level.

STEP 11

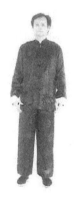

Step 11: Lower both arms to your side.

STEP 12

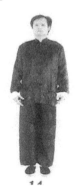

Step 12: Draw your left foot near your right (shoulder width apart) to close the form.

Form Five: Repulse Monkey

STEP 1

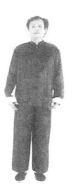

Step 1: Stand straight with feet slightly apart, knees unlocked, arms relaxed at the side of the body, and elbows slightly bent.

STEP 2

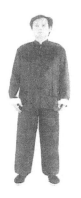

Step 2: Step slowly to your left with your left foot (toes touch down first, ending with feet spaced shoulder width apart).

STEP 3

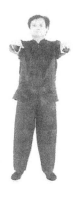

Step 3: Slowly raise both arms, with the elbows slightly bent, to shoulder height, wrists relaxed, hands dropped.

STEP 4

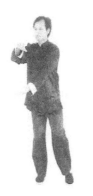

Step 4: Gradually shift your body weight to the right while dropping your left arm across your torso to the right to have both palms face each other to form the first "hold the ball" position (beach ball size) on the right.

STEP 5

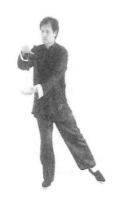

Step 5: Take a slow and comfortable step backwards to your left (diagonally at about 45 degrees) to land with the toes first.

STEP 6

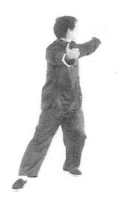

Step 6: Slowly shift your weight backwards onto your left leg. From here, rotate your trunk to the left (eyes follow the trunk rotation); simultaneously, push your right arm forward (palm faces out) while your left arm swings down past your left hip and then up to shoulder height (check: both palms now face up).

STEP 7

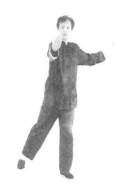

Step 7: Now, take a slow and comfortable step backwards to your right (diagonally at about 45 degrees) to land with the toes first.

STEP 8

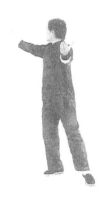

Step 8: Slowly rotate your trunk to the right (eyes follow the trunk rotation) and push your left arm forward (palm faces out) while your right arm swings down past your right hip and then up to shoulder height (check: both palms face up).

STEP 9

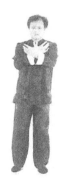

Step 9: Your rear (right) foot now moves forward to join your left foot, and both arms come together to cross at the wrists in front of your chest (check: your body weight is now centered).

STEP 10

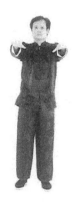

Step 10: Extend both arms forward, allowing them to separate (check: palms face down) at shoulder level.

STEP 11

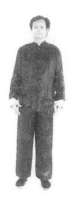

Step 11: Lower both arms to your side.

STEP 12

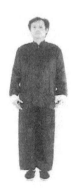

Step 12: Draw your left foot near your right (shoulder width apart) to close the form.

Form Six: Brush Knees

STEP 1

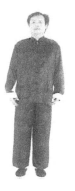

Step 1: Stand straight with feet slightly apart, knees unlocked, arms relaxed at the side of the body, and elbows slightly bent.

STEP 2

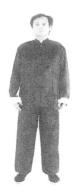

Step 2: Step slowly to your left with your left foot (toes touch down first, ending with feet spaced shoulder width apart).

STEP 3

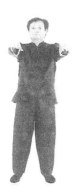

Step 3: Slowly raise both arms, with the elbows slightly bent, to shoulder height, wrists relaxed, hands dropped.

STEP 4

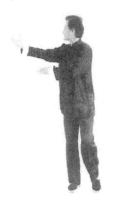

Step 4: Gradually shift your body weight to the right while dropping your left arm across your torso, and rotate your trunk slowly to the right with both arms swinging to the side; your right arm circles up to your ear level (palm faces up) and your left arm follows the same direction to the right (palm faces inward).

STEP 5

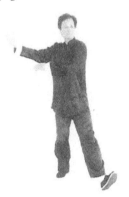

Step 5: Step with your left foot diagonally forward (at 45 degrees) to land on your left heel.

STEP 6

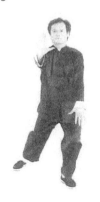

Step 6: Rotate your trunk to follow the direction of your left foot (weight gradually loads on your left leg); your right hand pushes directly forward (palm facing out) while your left hand sweeps down and across in front of the left knee (without touching).

STEP 7

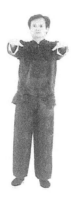

Step 7: Now, shift your weight backward onto your right leg, allowing your left heel to pivot (45 degrees) further to the left; swing and raise both arms to the left.

STEP 8

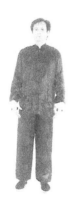

Step 8: Move your weight forward to the left leg and bring your right foot diagonally forward (about 45 degrees); simultaneously, bring both arms forward to cross your torso and allow your left hand to push directly forward (palm facing out); your right hand sweeps down and across in front of the right knee (without touching).

STEP 9

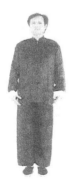

Step 9: Move your left foot forward to join the right foot. At the same time, bring both arms up to your chest level (hands crossed at the wrists) (check: your weight is now centered).

STEP 10

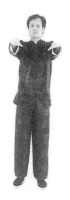

Step 10: Extend both arms forward, allowing them to separate (check: palms face down) at shoulder level.

STEP 11

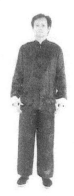

Step 11: Lower both arms to your side.

STEP 12

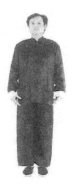

Step 12: Draw your left foot near your right (shoulder width apart) to close the form.

Form Seven: Fair Lady Works at Shuttles

STEP 1

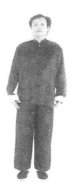

Step 1: Stand straight with feet slightly apart, knees unlocked, arms relaxed at the side of the body, and elbows slightly bent.

STEP 2

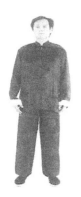

Step 2: Step slowly to your left with your left foot (toes touch down first, ending with feet spaced shoulder width apart).

STEP 3

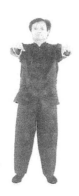

Step 3: Slowly raise both arms, with the elbows slightly bent, to shoulder height, wrists relaxed, hands dropped.

STEP 4

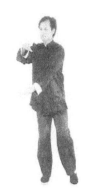

Step 4: Gradually shift your body weight to the right while dropping your left arm across your torso to the right to have both palms face each other to form the first "hold the ball" position (beach ball size) on the right.

STEP 5

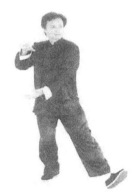

Step 5: With your left foot, take a diagonal step forward (about 45 degrees to your left) to land on your left heel.

STEP 6

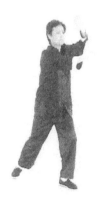

Step 6: Move your left hand upward (stopping slightly above your forehead) and then, with a slight trunk rotation to the left, turn your left palm outward while your right hand pushes straight forward (both palms face outward).

STEP 7

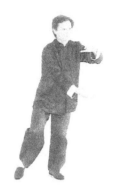

Step 7: Move your right leg next to the left leg and lower your right hand underneath your left hand (to form a "hold the ball" position) on the left.

STEP 8

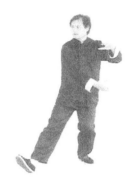

Step 8: With your right foot, take a diagonal step forward (about 45 degrees) to land on your right heel.

STEP 9

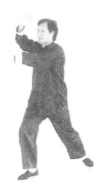

Step 9: As weight comes onto your right leg, your right hand moves upward (stopping slightly above your forehead) and then, with a slight trunk rotation to the right, turn your right palm outward while your left hand pushes diagonally forward (both palms face outward).

STEP 10

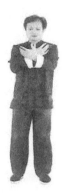

Step 10: Bring your left foot forward to join your right foot. At the same time, bring both arms up to your chest level (hands crossed at the wrists) (check: your weight is now centered).

STEP 11

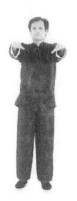

Step 11: Extend both arms forward allowing them to separate (check: palms face down) at shoulder level.

STEP 12

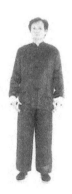

Step 12: Lower both arms to your side.

STEP 13

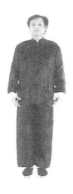

Step 13: Draw your left foot near your right (shoulder width apart) to close the form.

Form Eight: Grasp the Peacock's Tail

STEP 1

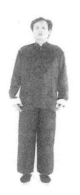

Step 1: Stand straight with feet slightly apart, knees unlocked, arms relaxed at the side of the body, and elbows slightly bent.

STEP 2

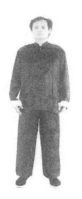

Step 2: Step slowly to your left with your left foot (toes touch down first, ending with feet spaced shoulder width apart).

STEP 3

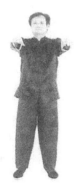

Step 3: Slowly raise both arms, with the elbows slightly bent, to shoulder height, wrists relaxed, hands dropped.

STEP 4

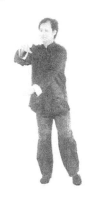

Step 4: Gradually shift your body weight to the right while dropping your left arm across your torso to the right to have both palms face each other to form the first "hold the ball" position (beach ball size) on the right. Now you are ready to perform the four movements: *Ward-off, Pull-back, Press, and Push*.

STEP 5

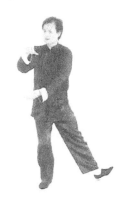

Step 5: *Ward-off:* From the ball-hold position, take a step to the left and slightly backward to land on your heel.

STEP 6

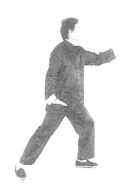

Step 6: Pivot outward on your left heel (rotate 90 degrees to the left) while simultaneously turning your waist toward the left. Along with the waist rotation, your left arm moves forward (to a blocking position – palm faces you); your right arm presses down obliquely to stop at your right hip (palm faces down).

STEP 7A

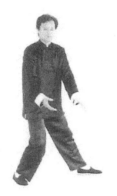

Step 7a: *Pull-back:* With a slight turn of your torso to the right, shift your weight backward and pull both hands back toward and across the right side of your body.

STEP 7B

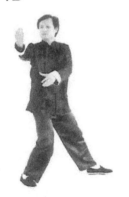

Step 7b: Continue your arm swing upwards with a semicircular motion, ending with your right arm facing your face on the side and your left arm in front of your chest (palm faces inward).

STEP 8

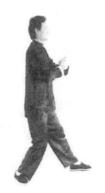

Step 8: Now, join your right hand to the left hand by placing the right palm on the left wrist in front of the chest.

STEP 9

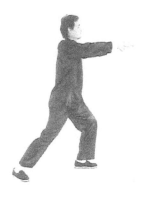

Step 9: *Press:* Press forward with both hands (touched at the wrists) until your arms are fully extended and hands are naturally separated.

STEP 10A

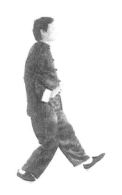

Step 10a: *Push:* Shift weight to the right leg as you pull both arms towards the body and down to stop at the waist (palms face forward) (with your left toes up).

STEP 10B

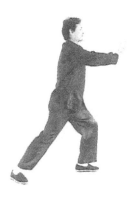

Step 10b: Now, push both arms out and forward (palms face forward) and up to shoulder level.

STEP 11

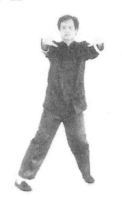

Step 11: Shift weight back onto right foot as you pivot your left heel and rotate your trunk 90 degrees to face the front along with both your arms, palms down, at shoulder level.

STEP 12

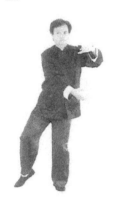

Step 12: Move your weight to your left leg, drop your right arm to form the ball-hold position on your left.

Now you repeat the movements for Ward-off, Push-back, Press, and Push on your right side.

STEP 13

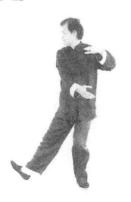

Step 13: *Ward-off:* Take a step to the right and slightly backward to land on your heel.

STEP 14

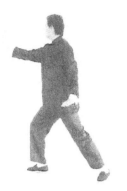

Step 14: Pivot outward on your right heel (rotate 90 degrees to the right) while simultaneously turning your waist toward the right. Along with the waist rotation, your right arm moves forward (to a blocking position– palm faces you); your left arm presses down obliquely to stop at your left hip (palm faces down).

STEP 15A

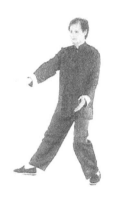

Step 15a: *Pull-back:* With a slight turn of your torso to the left, shift your weight backward and pull both hands back toward and across the left side of your body.

STEP 15B

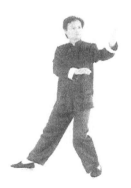

Step 15b: Continue your arm swing upwards with a semicircular motion, ending with your left arm facing your face on the side and your right arm in front of your chest (palm faces inward).

STEP 16

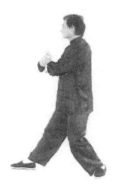

Step 16: Now, join your left hand to the right hand by placing the left palm on the right wrist in front of the chest.

STEP 17

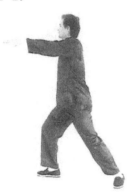

Step 17: *Press:* Press forward with both hands (touched at the wrists) until your arms are fully extended and hands are naturally separated.

STEP 18A

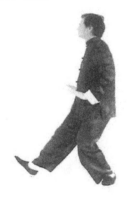

Step 18a: *Push:* Shift weight to the back as you pull both arms towards the body and down to stop at the waist (palms face forward) (toes up).

STEP 18B

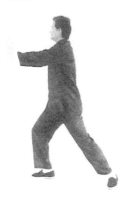

Step 18b: Now, shift weight forward as you push both arms out and up (palms face forward).

STEP 19

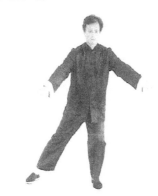

Step 19: Pivot on your right heel and rotate your trunk 90 degrees to face the front along with both your arms at shoulder level.

STEP 20

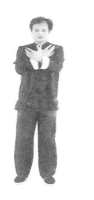

Step 20: Bring your right foot forward to join your left foot; simultaneously, bring both arms together to cross at the wrists in front of your chest (check: your body weight is now centered).

STEP 21

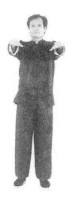

Step 21: Extend both arms forward allowing them to separate (check: palms face down) at shoulder level.

STEP 22

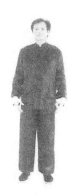

Step 22: Lower both arms to your side.

STEP 23

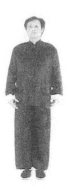

Step 23: Draw your left foot near your right (shoulder width apart) to close the form.

Put it All Together and Make it Flow

Congratulations! You have completed all eight individual forms. Now you might wonder how they can be all linked together to form a continuous flowing movement. As a visual aide, the next series of pictures links each movement of each form in sequence. We encourage you to follow the demonstration tape in addition to your class instruction to learn to perform the sequence.[33,34]

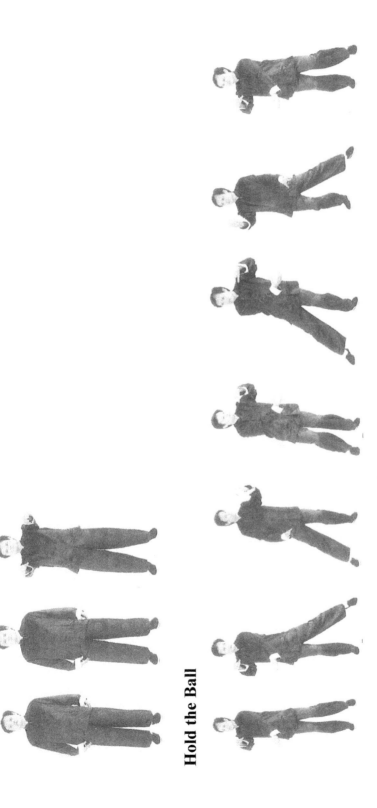

REVISED 07/18

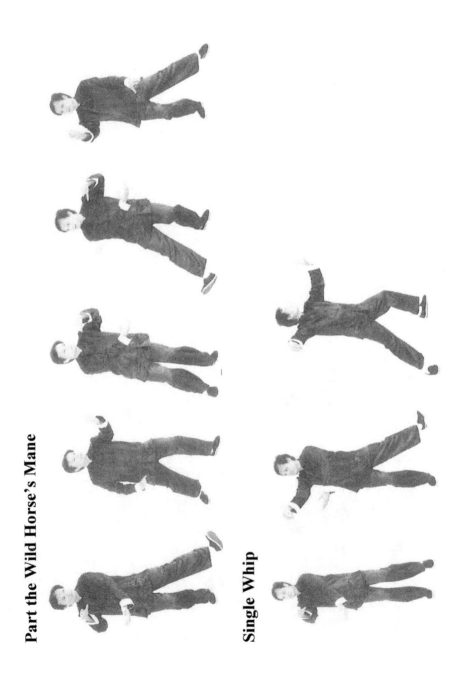

Part the Wild Horse's Mane

Single Whip

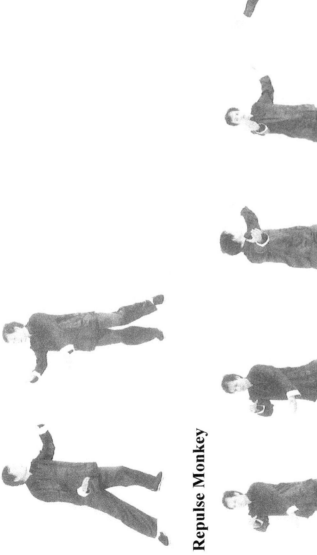

Wave Hands like Clouds

Repulse Monkey

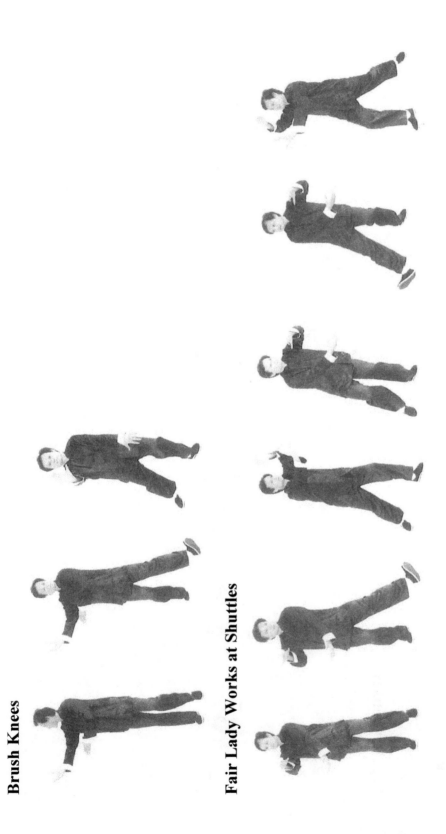

Brush Knees

Fair Lady Works at Shuttles

Grasp the Peacock's Tail

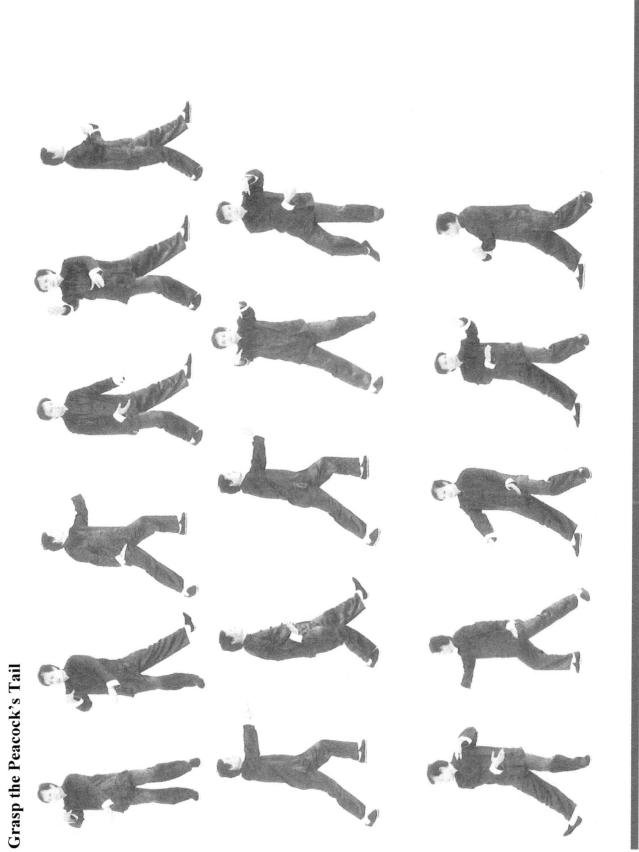

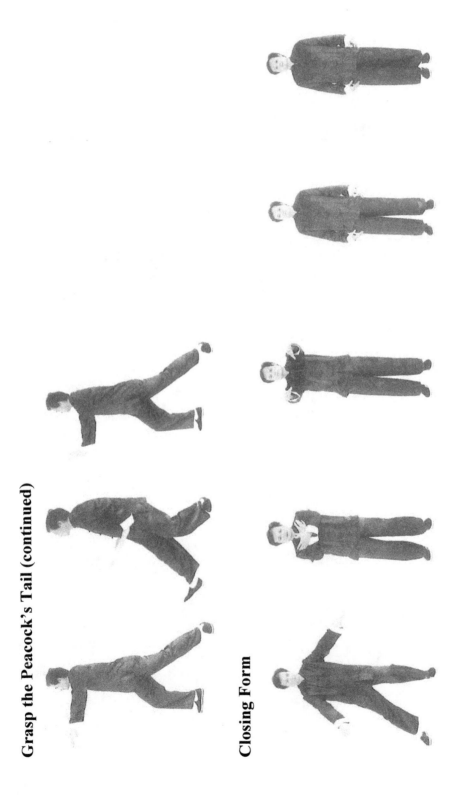

Grasp the Peacock's Tail (continued)

Closing Form

Key Resources

1. Li F, Harmer P, Fisher KJ, McAuley E, Chaumeton N, Eckstrom E, et al. Tai chi and fall reductions in older adults: a randomized controlled trial. J Gerontol A Biol Sci Med Sci 2005; 60(2):187-194.
2. Rubenstein L. Falls in older people: epidemiology, risk factors and strategies for prevention. Age and Ageing 2006;35(S2):ii37-ii41.
3. Centers for Disease Control and Prevention. Simply Put [online]. 2009. [cited 2011 Aug 21]. Available from URL: http://www.cdc.gov/healthliteracy/pdf/Simply_Put.pdf.
4. Kuramoto AM. Therapeutic benefits of tai chi exercise: research review. WMJ 2006;105(7):42-46.
5. Wang C, Schmid CH, Hibberd PL, Kalish R, Roubenoff R, Rones R, et al. Tai chi for treating knee osteoarthritis: designing a long-term follow up randomized controlled trial. BMC Musculoskelet Disord 2008;9(108).
6. Wolf SL, Barnhart HX, Kutner NG, McNeely E, Coogler C, Xu T. Reducing frailty and falls in older persons: An investigation of Tai Chi and computerized balance training. Journal of the American Geriatrics Society 1996 May;44(5):489-97.
7. Choi JH, Moon JS, & Song R. Effects of sun-style tai chi exercise on physical fitness and fall prevention in fall-prone older adults. J Adv Nurs 2005;51(2):150-157.
8. Kerr C. Translating "mind-in-body": two models of patient experience underlying a randomized controlled trial of qigong. Cult Med Psychiatry 2002;26(4):419-447.
9. Yeh GY, Wood MJ, Lorell BH, Stevenson LW, Eisenberg DM, Wayne PM, et al. Effects of tai chi mind-body movement therapy on functional status and exercise capacity in patients with chronic heart failure: a randomized controlled trial. Am J Med 2004;117(8):541-548.
10. Harmer PA, & Li, F. Tai Chi and falls prevention in older people. Med Sport Sci 2008;52:124-134.
11. Logghe I, Verhagen AP, Rademaker A, Zeeuwe P, Bierma-Zeinstra S, Van Rossum E, et al. Explaining the ineffectiveness of a tai chi fall prevention training for community-living older people: A process evaluation alongside a randomized clinical trial (RCT). Archives of Gerontology and Geriatrics 2011;52(3):357-362.
12. Sherrington C, Tiedemann A, Fairhall N, Close JCT, & Lord SR. Exercise to prevent falls in older adults: an updated meta-analysis and best practice recommendations. New South Wales Public Health Bulletin 2011;22(4):78-83
13. Wolf SL, O'Grady M, Easley KA, Guo Y, Kressig RW, & Kutner M. The influence of intense tai chi training on physical performance and hemodynamic outcomes in transitionally frail, older adults. J Gerontol A Biol Sci Med Sci 2006;61(2):184-189.

14. Logghe IH, Verhagen AP, Rademaker AC, Bierma-Zeinstra SM, van Rossum E, Faber MJ, et al. The effects of tai chi on fall prevention, fear of falling and balance in older people: a meta-analysis. Prev Med 2010;51(3-4):222-227.
15. Wolfson L, Whipple R, Derby C, Judge J, King M, Amerman P, et al. Balance and strength training in older adults: intervention gains and tai chi maintenance. J Am Geriatr Soc 1996;44(5):498-506
16. Li F, Harmer P, Mack KA, et al. Tai chi: moving for better balance – development of a community-based fall prevention program. J Phys Act Health 2008;5:445-455.
17. Oregon Research Institute. Tai chi: moving for better balance community implementation plan. 2008.
18. Li F, Harmer P, Glasgow R, Mack KA, Sleet D, Fisher KJ, et al. Translation of an effective tai chi intervention into a community-based falls-prevention program. Am J Public Health 2008;98(7):1195-1198.
19. Personal communication with Fuzhong Li, PhD, Portland OR, 2010 Oct.
20. Taylor-Davis S, Smiciklas-Wright H, Davis AC, Jensen GL, & Mitchell DC. Time and cost for recruiting older adults. J Am Geriatr Soc 1998;46(6):753-757.
21. Coleman EA, Tyll L, LaCroix AZ, Allen C, Leveille SG, Wallace JI, et al. Recruiting African-American older adults for a community-based health promotion intervention: which strategies are effective? Am J Prev Med 1997;13(6 Suppl):51-56.
22. Gitlin LN, Burgh D, Dodson C, & Freda M. Strategies to recruit older adults for participation in rehabilitation research. Topics in Geriatric Rehabilitation 195;11(1):10-19.
23. Centers for Disease Control and Prevention. Preventing Falls: How to Develop Community-based Fall Prevention Programs for Older Adults. 2008.
24. State of California Department of Public Health, Safe and Active Communities Branch, State and Local Injury Control Section. Tai chi: Moving For Better Balance Site Application. 2010.
25. State of California Department of Public Health, Safe and Active Communities Branch, State and Local Injury Control Section. Tai chi: Moving For Better Balance Instructor Agreement. 2010.
26. State of Oregon Health Authority, Office of Disease Prevention and Epidemiology, Injury and Violence Prevention Program. Tai chi Participant Registration Form. 2010.
27. State of Oregon Health Authority, Office of Disease Prevention and Epidemiology, Injury and Violence Prevention Program. Tai chi: Moving for Better Balance Class Observation Tool. 2010.
28. Oregon Research Institute. Tai chi: Moving for Better Balance Instructor Training Workshop, v1.2. Oregon Research Institute. 2009.
29. Jones CJ, Rikli RE, Beam WC. A 30-s chair-stand test as a measure of lower body strength in community-residing older adults. Res Q Exerc Sport. 1999 Jun;70(2):113-9.
30. Podsiadlo D, Richardson S. The timed "up and go": a test of basic functional mobility for frail elderly persons. JAGS 1991;39:142-148.
31. Rossiter-Fornoff JE, Wolfe SL, Wolfson L, Buchner DM. FICSIT Group. A cross-sectional validation study of the FICSIT common data base static balance measures. J Gerontol A Biol Sci Med Sci 1995;50A(6):M291–M297.
32. State of California Department of Public Health, Safe and Active Communities Branch, State and Local Injury Control Section. Tai chi: Moving for Better Balance *Peer Review Checklist*. 2010.
33. Oregon Research Institute. Tai chi: Moving for Better Balance Step-by-Step Guide. 2009.
34. Oregon Research Institute. Tai chi: Moving for Better Balance Guidebook. 2009.

Printed in the USA
CPSIA information can be obtained
at www.ICGtesting.com
LVHW011608071123
763300LV00016B/783